2025 SUPER EASY ANTI-INFLAMMATORY DIET FOR BEGINNERS WITH PICTURES

SAVANNAH STEELE

2025 SUPER EASY ANTI-INFLAMMATORY DIET FOR BEGINNERS WITH PICTURES

DAPEN

CONTENTS

Print ISBN: 978-1-0670770-4-4
E-book ISBN: 978-1-0670770-3-7
Publisher: Dapen Pubs

First Printing, 2025

INTRODUCTION

You're here because something's not right. Maybe you're dealing with chronic pain, fatigue, or bloating. Maybe you've been told that your inflammation levels are high and that it's causing health problems you just can't ignore. Or maybe you've tried diet after diet with little to no results. Sound familiar? If so, an anti-inflammatory diet could be exactly what you need — and this book is your guide to making it happen.

Why an Anti-Inflammatory Diet?

The truth is, inflammation is at the root of a lot of the health issues we struggle with today. Whether it's joint pain, weight gain, skin issues, or digestive problems, inflammation can cause a lot of damage over time. And, unfortunately, many of the foods we eat every day — sugar, processed carbs, refined oils — are the very things that fuel inflammation. If you've been feeling stuck or frustrated, it's because what you've been eating is likely making things worse.

This diet is about getting rid of the foods that keep your body in a constant state of inflammation and replacing them with real, nourishing ingredients that help heal and restore. By focusing on anti-inflammatory foods, you're not just "eating healthier" — you're helping your body get back to balance.

The Benefits of Reducing Inflammation

When you reduce inflammation, you start to feel better. It's that simple. But the benefits go beyond just feeling good in the moment. Lower inflammation means clearer skin, more energy, less joint pain, and even better sleep. It means supporting your immune system so that you can fight off illness more effectively. And in the long run, it's about reducing your risk for chronic diseases like heart disease, diabetes, and even cancer.

This isn't just about treating symptoms; it's about healing your body from the inside out. And when you do that, you'll be amazed at how much better you feel, both physically and mentally.

How This Book Helps You: Simple, Visual, and Beginner-Friendly

If you've never followed an anti-inflammatory diet before, it can seem overwhelming at first. But that's where this book comes in. I've designed it to be simple, practical, and visual — because I know that when you see exactly how something works, it's a lot easier to follow through. You don't need to be a master chef to benefit from this diet. You just need to be ready to make small, manageable changes, and this book will show you exactly how to do that.

I've broken everything down for you in a way that's easy to understand. No complicated recipes, no long shopping lists, and no fancy kitchen gadgets required. Whether you're brand new to cooking or you've been at it for years, this book will walk you through everything you need to know.

Essential Anti-Inflammatory Ingredients and Pantry Staples

One of the best parts about this way of eating is that it doesn't require a ton of expensive or hard-to-find ingredients. Many of the foods you'll need are already sitting in your pantry or local grocery store. We're talking about things like olive oil, turmeric, ginger, garlic, and a wide variety of fresh vegetables and fruits. These are the ingredients that will help you fight inflammation and promote healing.

In the next chapter, we'll dive into what foods you should be stocking up on and which ones to avoid at all costs. But first, just know that you're not alone in this journey. Reducing inflammation through food is one of the most powerful ways to take control of your health, and with this book, you've got a clear path forward.

CHAPTER 1

GETTING STARTED WITH EASE

So, you're ready to start reducing inflammation and feeling better. That's awesome! I get it — sometimes the idea of changing how we eat can feel a little overwhelming, especially when we're not sure where to start. But don't worry. I'm here to walk you through everything step-by-step, and we're keeping it simple. No need to complicate things. Just a few key changes and a little time is all it takes.

Understanding Inflammation and How Food Affects It

Let's start with the basics. Inflammation is your body's natural response to injury or infection. In small doses, it's actually a good thing — it's your immune system doing its job to protect you. But when inflammation sticks around too long (which happens if we keep eating the wrong things), it can lead to chronic issues like joint pain, weight gain, digestive problems, and even more serious conditions like heart disease and diabetes.

The foods you eat can either fuel this chronic inflammation or help calm it down. When we eat highly processed foods, sugars, and refined carbs, we're giving our body constant fuel for that fire. On the flip side, when we focus on whole, nutrient-rich foods like vegetables, healthy fats, and lean proteins, we're helping to put that fire out.

It's not about completely overhauling everything at once — it's about understanding how food works in your body and making small, smart choices. Once you start swapping out those inflammatory foods and replacing them with anti-inflammatory ones, you'll start to feel the difference.

Foods to Enjoy and Foods to Avoid

Here's the thing: you don't need to worry about a complicated list of foods to avoid forever. All you need to know is that the anti-inflammatory diet is based on whole, nourishing foods that your body thrives on. You can still enjoy delicious meals that make you feel good. But there are some foods you need to leave behind, at least for a while.

Foods to Enjoy:

- **Leafy Greens**: Kale, spinach, arugula — these veggies are packed with antioxidants and can help reduce inflammation.
- **Berries**: Blueberries, strawberries, and raspberries are loaded with vitamins and antioxidants that fight inflammation.
- **Fatty Fish**: Salmon, mackerel, sardines — these are rich in omega-3 fatty acids, which are your body's best friends when it comes to lowering inflammation.
- **Nuts and Seeds**: Walnuts, almonds, flaxseeds, chia seeds — these contain healthy fats and fiber that help keep inflammation in check.
- **Olive Oil**: Packed with healthy fats, it's a great addition to your meals and can help reduce inflammation in your body.

- **Turmeric and Ginger**: These are natural anti-inflammatory powerhouses. Use them in your cooking or even in teas for an extra healing boost.

Foods to Avoid:

- **Processed Foods**: Anything that's packaged, loaded with sugar, preservatives, and artificial ingredients. This includes most packaged snacks, frozen meals, and fast food.
- **Refined Carbs**: White bread, pastries, and other products made with white flour cause blood sugar spikes that fuel inflammation.
- **Sugar**: I'm talking about added sugars — soda, candy, sweetened coffee, and baked goods. These are a huge driver of inflammation and should be minimized.
- **Seed Oils**: Vegetable, canola, and soybean oils are high in omega-6 fatty acids, which can promote inflammation when consumed in excess.

Meal Planning Made Simple

Now that you know which foods to focus on and which ones to avoid, it's time to make meal planning easy. The secret? Keep it simple and stick to the basics.

Here's how you can make meal planning easier:

1. **Pick Your Protein**: Start with a lean protein like chicken, turkey, salmon, or plant-based options like beans and lentils.
2. **Choose Your Veggies**: Aim for a variety of colorful vegetables, especially greens like spinach, kale, or broccoli.
3. **Add Healthy Fats**: Include things like olive oil, avocado, or a handful of nuts to your meals for added flavor and anti-inflammatory benefits.

4. **Keep Grains Minimal**: When you do include grains, opt for whole grains like quinoa or brown rice. But keep your focus on veggies.
5. **Batch Cook**: Cook in larger quantities so you can easily assemble meals throughout the week.

Planning doesn't have to be difficult. Just pick a few things you like, and make sure they're available when you're hungry.

Tips for Cooking for Beginners (With Pictures)

When you're just getting started with cooking, it's easy to feel like you don't know where to begin. But cooking for an anti-inflammatory diet is easier than it sounds. Here are a few simple tips to get you in the kitchen and feeling confident:

- **Start with One Pan Meals**: Keep it simple by roasting vegetables and protein on a sheet pan. You'll have a complete meal with minimal clean-up.
- **Prep Ahead**: Chop vegetables, marinate proteins, or make large batches of things like soups and salads. Having prepped ingredients makes meals come together faster.
- **Use Simple Seasonings**: Stick to a few key spices — garlic, turmeric, ginger, rosemary, and thyme — to add flavor without extra effort.
- **Try the Slow Cooker or Instant Pot**: These tools take the guesswork out of cooking. Just throw in your ingredients and let them cook while you go about your day.

With the right tools and a little practice, you'll start to feel more at ease in the kitchen. Don't be afraid to experiment with new flavors and textures. Anti-inflammatory eating can be delicious and satisfying.

CHAPTER

2

QUICK AND HEALING BREAKFASTS

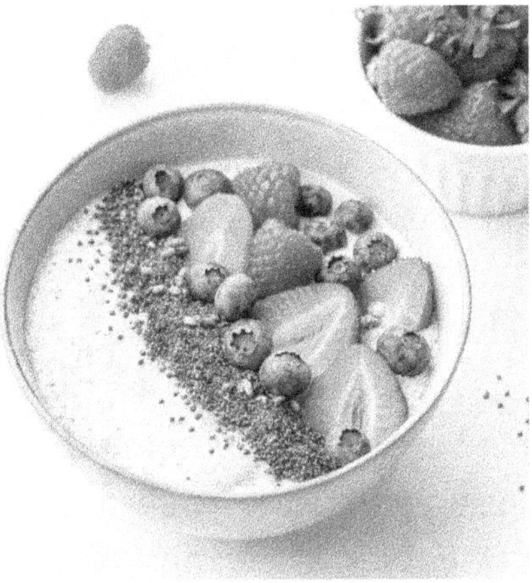

Overnight Chia Pudding with Berries

This easy and nutritious breakfast is a great way to start your day on the right foot. Packed with fiber, antioxidants, and healthy fats, this chia pudding is perfect for fighting inflammation while keeping you full and satisfied. Top with fresh berries for an added anti-inflammatory boost.

Recipe Details:

- **Servings:** 2
- **Prep Time:** 10 minutes
- **Cook Time:** 0 minutes (overnight soak)
- **Difficulty Level:** Easy
- **Dietary Notes:** Gluten-free, dairy-free, vegan, high in omega-3s, anti-inflammatory

Ingredients:

- 1/2 cup chia seeds
- 1 cup almond milk (or other non-dairy milk)

- 1 tablespoon maple syrup (optional)
- 1/2 teaspoon vanilla extract
- 1/2 cup mixed berries (blueberries, strawberries, raspberries)
- 1 tablespoon almond butter (optional for extra richness)

Step-by-Step Instructions:

1. In a medium bowl or jar, combine the chia seeds, almond milk, maple syrup (if using), and vanilla extract. Stir well to ensure the chia seeds are evenly distributed.
2. Cover the bowl or jar and refrigerate overnight, or for at least 4 hours, to allow the chia seeds to soak and expand.
3. Once ready, give the pudding a good stir to break up any clumps.
4. Divide the pudding into two servings and top with fresh berries and a spoonful of almond butter, if desired.
5. Enjoy your anti-inflammatory breakfast!

Tips and Variations:

- **Substitution:** Use coconut milk or oat milk for a creamier consistency.
- **Pairing Idea:** Serve with a warm cup of green tea for an added anti-inflammatory boost.
- **Variation:** Add a sprinkle of cinnamon or turmeric for extra flavor and inflammation-fighting benefits.

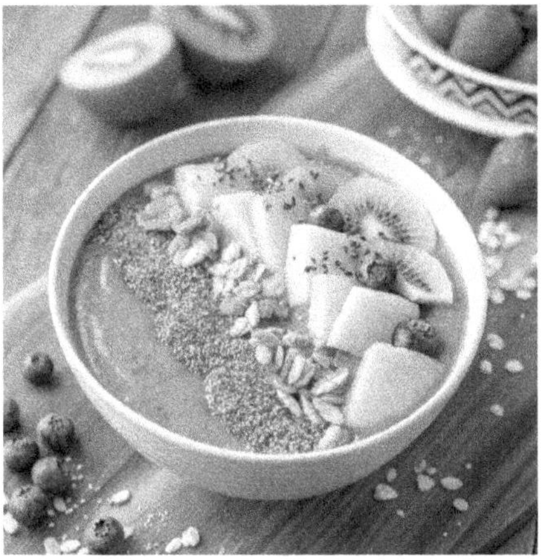

Anti-Inflammatory Smoothie Bowl

This vibrant smoothie bowl is packed with nutrient-dense ingredients that support a healthy, inflammation-free body. With spinach, turmeric, and frozen berries, it's the perfect way to power up your morning with antioxidants and fiber.

Recipe Details:

- **Servings:** 1
- **Prep Time:** 5 minutes
- **Cook Time:** 0 minutes
- **Difficulty Level:** Easy
- **Dietary Notes:** Gluten-free, dairy-free, vegan, anti-inflammatory, high in fiber

Ingredients:

- 1/2 cup frozen mixed berries
- 1/2 cup fresh spinach
- 1/4 cup almond milk (or other non-dairy milk)

- 1/2 teaspoon ground turmeric
- 1 tablespoon flaxseeds
- 1/2 banana
- 1 tablespoon chia seeds
- Toppings: sliced almonds, fresh berries, and shredded coconut

Step-by-Step Instructions:

1. In a blender, combine the frozen berries, spinach, almond milk, turmeric, flaxseeds, banana, and chia seeds.
2. Blend until smooth and thick. Add more almond milk if needed to reach the desired consistency.
3. Pour into a bowl and top with sliced almonds, fresh berries, and shredded coconut.
4. Enjoy your anti-inflammatory smoothie bowl!

Tips and Variations:

- **Substitution:** Use frozen mango or pineapple for a tropical twist.
- **Pairing Idea:** This smoothie bowl pairs wonderfully with a handful of walnuts for an added omega-3 boost.
- **Variation:** For added protein, toss in a scoop of plant-based protein powder.

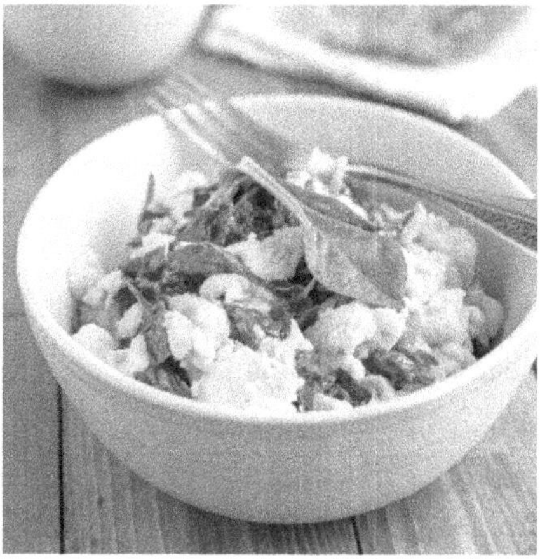

Turmeric Scrambled Eggs with Spinach

This hearty breakfast features anti-inflammatory turmeric and spinach, combined with fluffy scrambled eggs for a satisfying, nutritious meal. Perfect for starting the day with a protein-packed, inflammation-fighting dish.

Recipe Details:

- **Servings:** 2
- **Prep Time:** 5 minutes
- **Cook Time:** 5 minutes
- **Difficulty Level:** Easy
- **Dietary Notes:** Gluten-free, high in protein, anti-inflammatory

Ingredients:

- 4 large eggs
- 1 tablespoon olive oil
- 1/2 teaspoon ground turmeric

- 1/2 cup fresh spinach, chopped
- Salt and pepper, to taste
- Optional: A pinch of cayenne pepper or paprika for extra flavor

Step-by-Step Instructions:

1. In a bowl, whisk the eggs with a pinch of salt, pepper, and turmeric until well combined.
2. Heat the olive oil in a non-stick pan over medium heat.
3. Add the egg mixture to the pan and cook, stirring occasionally, until the eggs are fully scrambled.
4. Just before the eggs are done, add the chopped spinach and cook for another minute, until wilted.
5. Serve warm with a sprinkle of cayenne or paprika, if desired.

Tips and Variations:

- **Substitution:** For a dairy-free version, you can add a splash of non-dairy milk to the egg mixture.
- **Pairing Idea:** Serve with a slice of whole-grain toast or avocado for extra fiber and healthy fats.
- **Variation:** Add sautéed mushrooms or onions for a heartier breakfast.

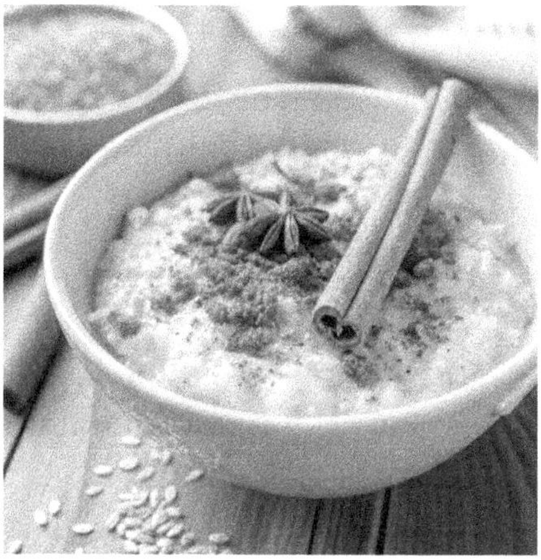

Oatmeal with Flaxseed and Warm Spices

A cozy, anti-inflammatory bowl of oatmeal is a perfect way to start the day. With the added benefits of flaxseed, cinnamon, and ginger, this warm breakfast will help soothe your body while providing fiber and healthy fats.

Recipe Details:

- **Servings:** 2
- **Prep Time:** 5 minutes
- **Cook Time:** 10 minutes
- **Difficulty Level:** Easy
- **Dietary Notes:** Gluten-free, high in fiber, anti-inflammatory, vegetarian

Ingredients:

- 1 cup rolled oats
- 2 cups water or almond milk
- 1 tablespoon flaxseed, ground

- 1/2 teaspoon cinnamon
- 1/4 teaspoon ground ginger
- 1 tablespoon maple syrup or honey (optional)
- Toppings: chopped nuts, fresh fruit, or coconut flakes

Step-by-Step Instructions:

1. In a medium pot, bring the water or almond milk to a boil.
2. Add the oats, reduce the heat, and simmer for about 5-7 minutes, stirring occasionally.
3. Stir in the ground flaxseed, cinnamon, and ginger, and cook for another 2-3 minutes until the oats reach your desired consistency.
4. Sweeten with maple syrup or honey, if desired.
5. Serve topped with fresh fruit, chopped nuts, or coconut flakes.

Tips and Variations:

- **Substitution:** Use chia seeds instead of flaxseed for added omega-3s.
- **Pairing Idea:** Pair this oatmeal with a cup of green tea to boost the anti-inflammatory benefits.
- **Variation:** Add a spoonful of almond butter for added richness and healthy fats.

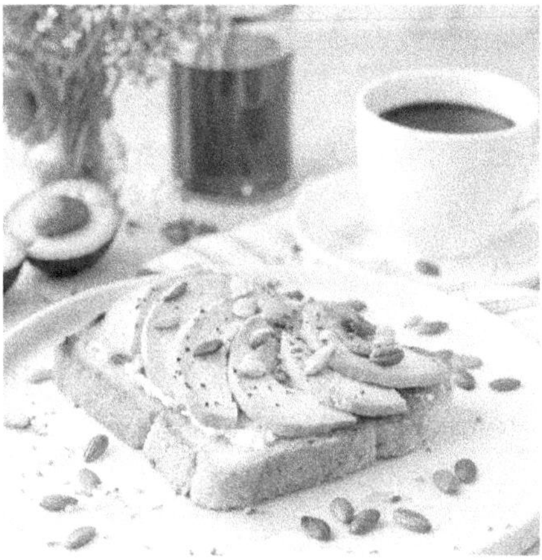

Avocado Toast with Olive Oil and Seeds

This simple yet nourishing breakfast features creamy avocado on whole-grain toast, drizzled with olive oil and sprinkled with anti-inflammatory seeds. It's an easy meal that's packed with healthy fats and fiber to start your day right.

Recipe Details:

- **Servings:** 2
- **Prep Time:** 5 minutes
- **Cook Time:** 5 minutes
- **Difficulty Level:** Easy
- **Dietary Notes:** Gluten-free (if using GF bread), dairy-free, high in healthy fats, anti-inflammatory

Ingredients:

- 2 slices whole-grain or gluten-free bread
- 1 ripe avocado
- 1 tablespoon extra virgin olive oil

- 1 tablespoon chia seeds
- 1 tablespoon sunflower seeds
- Salt and pepper, to taste
- Optional: Red pepper flakes for a spicy kick

Step-by-Step Instructions:

1. Toast the bread slices to your desired crispness.
2. While the bread is toasting, slice the avocado in half, remove the pit, and scoop out the flesh.
3. Mash the avocado with a fork and season with salt and pepper.
4. Spread the mashed avocado evenly over the toasted bread.
5. Drizzle with olive oil and sprinkle with chia seeds, sunflower seeds, and optional red pepper flakes.
6. Serve immediately and enjoy your anti-inflammatory breakfast.

Tips and Variations:

- **Substitution:** Use flaxseeds instead of chia seeds for a different texture.
- **Pairing Idea:** Add a poached egg on top for extra protein.
- **Variation:** Try adding a few slices of tomato or cucumber for extra flavor and crunch.

CHAPTER

3

NOURISHING LUNCHES IN NO TIME

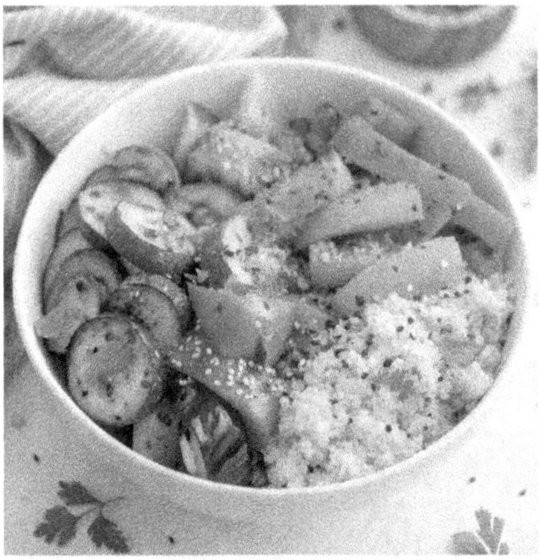

Quinoa and Roasted Veggie Power Bowl

This vibrant power bowl is packed with protein-rich quinoa, anti-inflammatory roasted veggies, and a simple lemon-tahini dressing that brings everything together. It's the perfect meal for a nourishing, feel-good lunch that's full of fiber and healthy fats.

Recipe Details:

- **Servings:** 2
- **Prep Time:** 10 minutes
- **Cook Time:** 25 minutes
- **Difficulty Level:** Easy
- **Dietary Notes:** Gluten-free, vegan, high in fiber, anti-inflammatory

Ingredients:

- 1/2 cup quinoa
- 1 cup water
- 1 zucchini, sliced

- 1 bell pepper, chopped
- 1/2 red onion, sliced
- 1 tablespoon olive oil
- 1/2 teaspoon ground turmeric
- Salt and pepper, to taste
- 1/4 cup hummus (for topping)
- Fresh parsley for garnish

For the Lemon-Tahini Dressing:

- 2 tablespoons tahini
- Juice of 1 lemon
- 1 tablespoon olive oil
- 1 teaspoon maple syrup (optional)
- Water to thin, as needed
- Salt, to taste

Step-by-Step Instructions:

1. Preheat your oven to 400°F (200°C).
2. Rinse the quinoa under cold water and combine it with 1 cup of water in a pot. Bring to a boil, then reduce the heat to low and cover. Cook for about 15 minutes, or until the water is absorbed and the quinoa is tender.
3. While the quinoa cooks, place the zucchini, bell pepper, and red onion on a baking sheet. Drizzle with olive oil, turmeric, salt, and pepper. Roast for 20-25 minutes, or until the vegetables are tender and lightly browned.
4. While the veggies roast, prepare the dressing. In a small bowl, whisk together tahini, lemon juice, olive oil, maple syrup, and salt. Add water to reach your desired consistency.

5. To assemble, divide the cooked quinoa between two bowls. Top with roasted veggies, a dollop of hummus, and a drizzle of lemon-tahini dressing. Garnish with fresh parsley.
6. Serve and enjoy!

Tips and Variations:

- **Substitution:** Add any seasonal veggies like sweet potatoes or Brussels sprouts for variety.
- **Pairing Idea:** Serve with a side of mixed greens for an even bigger nutrient boost.
- **Variation:** For added protein, top with a boiled egg or grilled chicken.

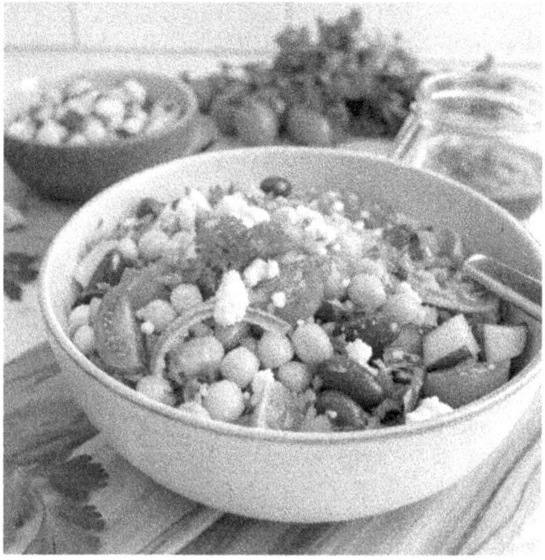

Mediterranean Chickpea Salad

This fresh and colorful Mediterranean Chickpea Salad is a perfect, no-cook lunch that's packed with antioxidants, healthy fats, and plant-based protein. It's perfect for reducing inflammation while keeping you full and energized.

Recipe Details:

- **Servings:** 2
- **Prep Time:** 10 minutes
- **Cook Time:** 0 minutes
- **Difficulty Level:** Easy
- **Dietary Notes:** Gluten-free, vegan, high in fiber, anti-inflammatory

Ingredients:

- 1 can (15 oz) chickpeas, drained and rinsed
- 1 cucumber, diced
- 1 cup cherry tomatoes, halved

- 1/4 red onion, finely chopped
- 1/4 cup Kalamata olives, sliced
- 1/4 cup feta cheese (optional)
- 2 tablespoons extra virgin olive oil
- Juice of 1 lemon
- 1 teaspoon dried oregano
- Salt and pepper, to taste

Step-by-Step Instructions:

1. In a large bowl, combine the chickpeas, cucumber, cherry tomatoes, red onion, olives, and feta (if using).
2. In a small bowl, whisk together the olive oil, lemon juice, oregano, salt, and pepper.
3. Pour the dressing over the salad and toss to combine.
4. Serve immediately or refrigerate for 30 minutes to let the flavors meld.
5. Enjoy!

Tips and Variations:

- **Substitution:** Use vegan feta or omit it for a fully plant-based meal.
- **Pairing Idea:** Serve with whole-grain pita or toasted bread for added fiber.
- **Variation:** Add a handful of chopped fresh parsley or mint for extra flavor.

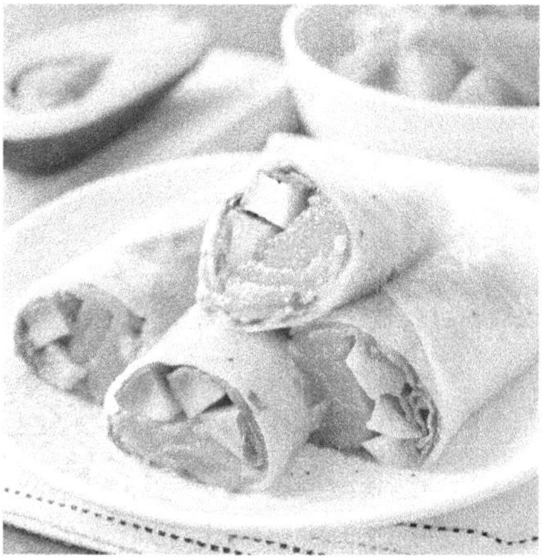

Salmon and Avocado Wraps

These delicious and filling wraps are made with flaky salmon, creamy avocado, and a crunchy veggie filling. They're quick to put together and loaded with anti-inflammatory omega-3 fatty acids, perfect for a healthy and satisfying lunch.

Recipe Details:

- **Servings:** 2
- **Prep Time:** 5 minutes
- **Cook Time:** 10 minutes (for salmon)
- **Difficulty Level:** Easy
- **Dietary Notes:** Gluten-free, dairy-free, high in omega-3s, anti-inflammatory

Ingredients:

- 2 small salmon fillets
- 1 tablespoon olive oil
- Salt and pepper, to taste

- 1 ripe avocado, sliced
- 2 large lettuce leaves (for wraps)
- 1/2 cup shredded carrots
- 1/4 cup cucumber, julienned
- 1 tablespoon fresh dill (optional)

Step-by-Step Instructions:

1. Heat the olive oil in a pan over medium-high heat. Season the salmon fillets with salt and pepper. Cook the salmon for 3-4 minutes per side, until fully cooked and flaky.
2. While the salmon cooks, prepare the veggie filling by combining the avocado slices, shredded carrots, cucumber, and dill (if using).
3. Once the salmon is cooked, break it into large flakes with a fork.
4. To assemble the wraps, lay the lettuce leaves flat, and top each with a portion of salmon and the avocado-veggie mixture.
5. Wrap the lettuce around the filling and serve immediately.
6. Enjoy your anti-inflammatory lunch!

Tips and Variations:

- **Substitution:** Swap the salmon for grilled chicken or tofu for a different protein.
- **Pairing Idea:** Serve with a side of quinoa or a mixed green salad for extra fiber.
- **Variation:** Add a drizzle of lemon juice or tahini for extra flavor.

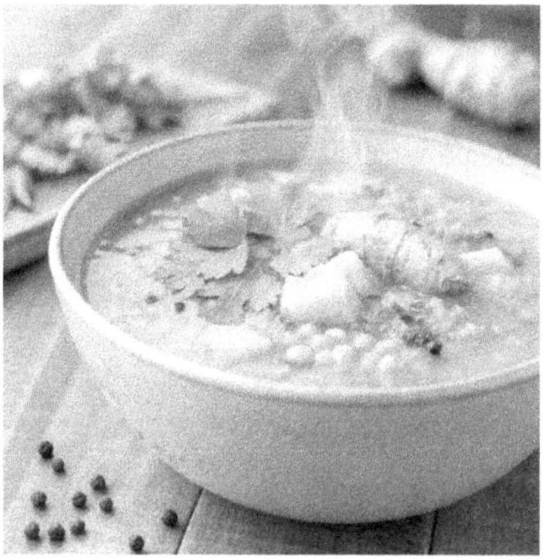

Lentil Soup with Turmeric and Ginger

This hearty, nourishing lentil soup is packed with flavor and anti-inflammatory goodness. With the warmth of turmeric and ginger, it's the perfect meal to soothe and heal, while being full of fiber and plant-based protein.

Recipe Details:

- **Servings:** 4
- **Prep Time:** 10 minutes
- **Cook Time:** 30 minutes
- **Difficulty Level:** Easy
- **Dietary Notes:** Vegan, gluten-free, high in fiber, anti-inflammatory

Ingredients:

- 1 tablespoon olive oil
- 1 onion, chopped
- 2 cloves garlic, minced

- 1 cup dried lentils, rinsed
- 1 teaspoon ground turmeric
- 1 teaspoon ground ginger
- 4 cups vegetable broth
- 1 can (15 oz) diced tomatoes
- Salt and pepper, to taste
- Fresh parsley, for garnish

Step-by-Step Instructions:

1. In a large pot, heat the olive oil over medium heat. Add the chopped onion and garlic, and sauté for 5 minutes until soft.
2. Add the lentils, turmeric, ginger, vegetable broth, and diced tomatoes to the pot. Bring to a boil, then reduce the heat to low and simmer for 25-30 minutes, or until the lentils are tender.
3. Season with salt and pepper to taste.
4. Serve warm, garnished with fresh parsley.
5. Enjoy this comforting, anti-inflammatory soup!

Tips and Variations:

- **Substitution:** Use yellow split peas instead of lentils for a variation in texture.
- **Pairing Idea:** Serve with whole-grain bread or a side salad for a complete meal.
- **Variation:** Add spinach or kale during the last 5 minutes of cooking for an extra dose of greens.

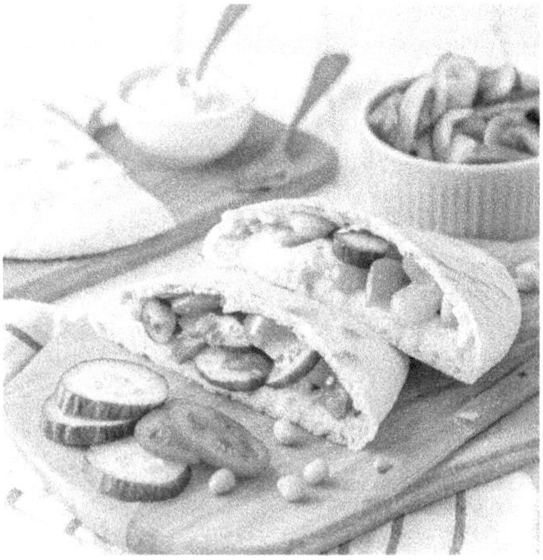

Hummus and Veggie-Stuffed Pita

This simple and satisfying pita is filled with creamy hummus, fresh veggies, and a tangy dressing. It's a light, anti-inflammatory meal that's perfect for a busy lunch when you want something healthy and easy.

Recipe Details:

- **Servings:** 2
- **Prep Time:** 5 minutes
- **Cook Time:** 0 minutes
- **Difficulty Level:** Easy
- **Dietary Notes:** Vegan, gluten-free (if using GF pita), anti-inflammatory

Ingredients:

- 2 whole wheat or gluten-free pita pockets
- 1/2 cup hummus
- 1 cucumber, thinly sliced

- 1 tomato, thinly sliced
- 1/4 red onion, thinly sliced
- 1/2 cup mixed greens
- 1 tablespoon olive oil
- Juice of 1/2 lemon
- Salt and pepper, to taste

Step-by-Step Instructions:

1. Slice the pita pockets in half to create two pockets.
2. Spread a generous layer of hummus inside each pita.
3. Stuff each pita with cucumber, tomato, onion, and mixed greens.
4. Drizzle with olive oil and lemon juice, then season with salt and pepper.
5. Serve immediately and enjoy!

Tips and Variations:

- **Substitution:** Use a dairy-free yogurt dressing instead of olive oil and lemon for a creamier texture.
- **Pairing Idea:** Serve with a side of roasted sweet potatoes for a nutrient-dense lunch.
- **Variation:** Add avocado slices for extra healthy fats and creaminess.

CHAPTER

4

COZY, HEALING DINNERS FOR TWO

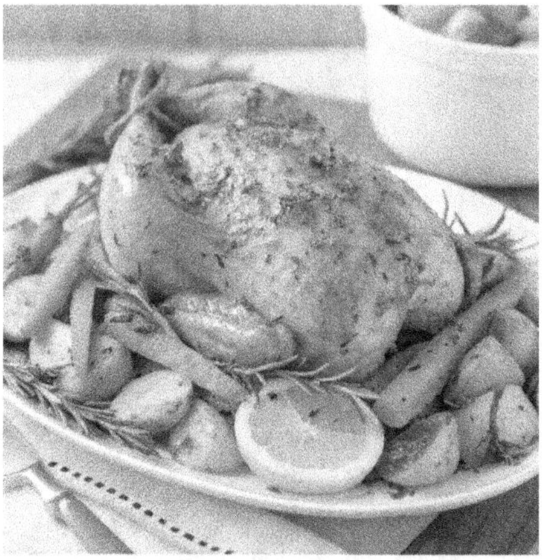

Baked Lemon Herb Chicken with Roasted Veggies

This simple yet flavorful baked chicken is marinated with lemon and herbs and paired with roasted veggies, making it the perfect cozy, anti-inflammatory dinner. The combination of lean protein and nutrient-rich vegetables ensures you get the best of both worlds in this easy-to-make meal.

Recipe Details:

- **Servings:** 2
- **Prep Time:** 10 minutes
- **Cook Time:** 35 minutes
- **Difficulty Level:** Easy
- **Dietary Notes:** Gluten-free, dairy-free, high in protein, anti-inflammatory

Ingredients:

- 2 boneless, skinless chicken breasts
- 1 lemon, zested and juiced

- 2 tablespoons olive oil
- 1 teaspoon dried rosemary
- 1 teaspoon dried thyme
- 2 cloves garlic, minced
- Salt and pepper, to taste
- 1 cup baby carrots
- 1 cup Brussels sprouts, halved
- 1 tablespoon olive oil (for veggies)

Step-by-Step Instructions:

1. Preheat your oven to 400°F (200°C).
2. In a small bowl, combine the lemon zest, lemon juice, olive oil, rosemary, thyme, garlic, salt, and pepper.
3. Place the chicken breasts in a resealable plastic bag or shallow dish and pour the marinade over the chicken. Let it marinate for at least 15 minutes.
4. While the chicken marinates, prepare the veggies. Toss the baby carrots and Brussels sprouts with olive oil, salt, and pepper, and spread them out on a baking sheet.
5. After the chicken has marinated, place it on a separate baking sheet or alongside the vegetables if there's room.
6. Roast the chicken and vegetables in the preheated oven for 25-30 minutes, or until the chicken reaches an internal temperature of 165°F (74°C) and the vegetables are tender and lightly caramelized.
7. Serve the chicken alongside the roasted veggies and enjoy a healing, flavorful meal.

Tips and Variations:

- **Substitution:** Use bone-in chicken thighs for a richer flavor and juicier result.

- **Pairing Idea:** Serve with a side of quinoa or brown rice for a fuller meal.
- **Variation:** Add other root vegetables like sweet potatoes or parsnips for more variety.

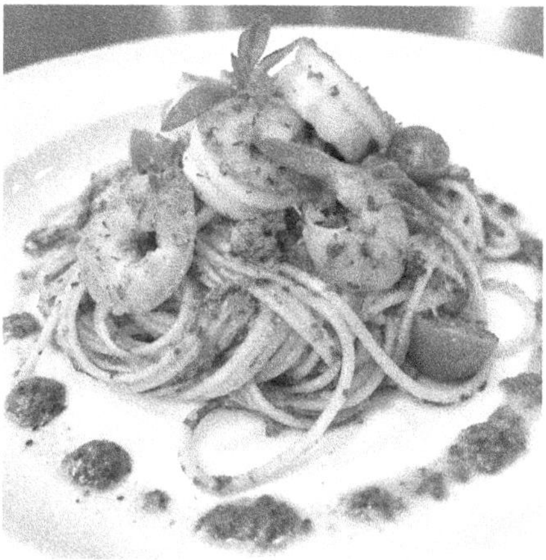

Zucchini Noodles with Pesto and Grilled Shrimp

Zucchini noodles (zoodles) make a healthy, low-carb alternative to pasta, while the pesto and grilled shrimp add flavor and protein to make this a light yet satisfying dinner. It's an anti-inflammatory dish that's easy to make and perfect for cozying up with after a long day.

Recipe Details:

- **Servings:** 2
- **Prep Time:** 10 minutes
- **Cook Time:** 10 minutes
- **Difficulty Level:** Easy
- **Dietary Notes:** Gluten-free, dairy-free (if using vegan pesto), high in protein, anti-inflammatory

Ingredients:

- 2 medium zucchinis, spiralized
- 1/2 lb (225g) shrimp, peeled and deveined

- 1 tablespoon olive oil (for shrimp)
- Salt and pepper, to taste

For the Pesto:

- 1/4 cup fresh basil leaves
- 2 tablespoons pine nuts
- 1/4 cup olive oil
- 2 cloves garlic
- 1 tablespoon nutritional yeast (or Parmesan if not dairy-free)
- Salt and pepper, to taste

Step-by-Step Instructions:

1. To make the pesto, combine basil, pine nuts, olive oil, garlic, nutritional yeast, salt, and pepper in a food processor. Blend until smooth, adding more olive oil if necessary to reach desired consistency.
2. Heat the olive oil in a grill pan or skillet over medium heat. Season the shrimp with salt and pepper, then cook for 2-3 minutes on each side, until they are pink and opaque.
3. In a separate pan, sauté the zucchini noodles over medium heat for 2-3 minutes, just until tender (don't overcook, or they'll become soggy).
4. Toss the zoodles with the pesto until they're well coated.
5. Serve the zucchini noodles topped with grilled shrimp and a drizzle of extra pesto.

Tips and Variations:

- **Substitution:** Swap the shrimp for grilled chicken or tofu for a vegetarian version.

- **Pairing Idea:** Serve with a side of roasted vegetables or a fresh salad.
- **Variation:** Add a handful of sun-dried tomatoes for extra depth of flavor.

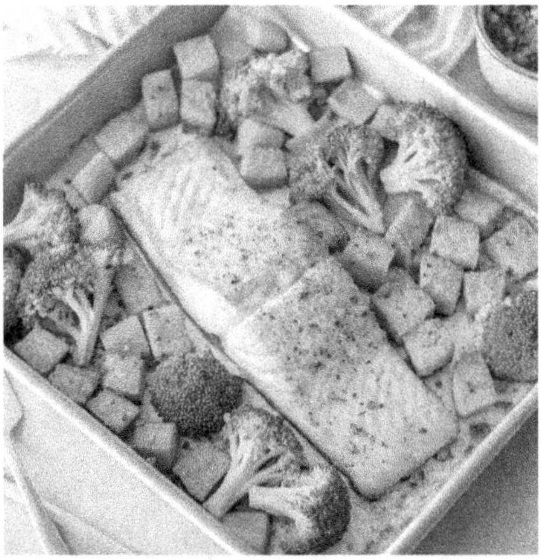

Sheet Pan Salmon with Sweet Potatoes and Broccoli

This sheet pan dinner is the perfect balance of healthy fats, protein, and fiber. The salmon is rich in omega-3 fatty acids, while the roasted sweet potatoes and broccoli provide a hearty, anti-inflammatory base. It's a simple, one-pan meal that's perfect for a cozy dinner with minimal cleanup.

Recipe Details:

- **Servings:** 2
- **Prep Time:** 10 minutes
- **Cook Time:** 30 minutes
- **Difficulty Level:** Easy
- **Dietary Notes:** Gluten-free, dairy-free, high in omega-3s, anti-inflammatory

Ingredients:

- 2 salmon fillets (6 oz each)

- 1 medium sweet potato, cubed
- 1 cup broccoli florets
- 2 tablespoons olive oil
- 1 teaspoon smoked paprika
- 1 teaspoon garlic powder
- Salt and pepper, to taste
- Lemon wedges for serving

Step-by-Step Instructions:

1. Preheat your oven to 400°F (200°C).
2. On a large sheet pan, toss the cubed sweet potatoes with 1 tablespoon of olive oil, smoked paprika, garlic powder, salt, and pepper. Spread them in a single layer.
3. Roast the sweet potatoes in the preheated oven for 15 minutes.
4. While the sweet potatoes are roasting, prepare the salmon. Drizzle with the remaining tablespoon of olive oil and season with salt and pepper.
5. After the sweet potatoes have roasted for 15 minutes, add the salmon fillets and broccoli to the sheet pan.
6. Roast for an additional 12-15 minutes, until the salmon is cooked through and flakes easily with a fork, and the broccoli is tender.
7. Serve the salmon, sweet potatoes, and broccoli with a wedge of lemon for extra flavor.

Tips and Variations:

- **Substitution:** Swap the salmon for another fatty fish like mackerel or trout.
- **Pairing Idea:** Serve with a side of quinoa or wild rice for extra fiber.

- **Variation:** Add a sprinkle of crushed red pepper flakes for a little heat.

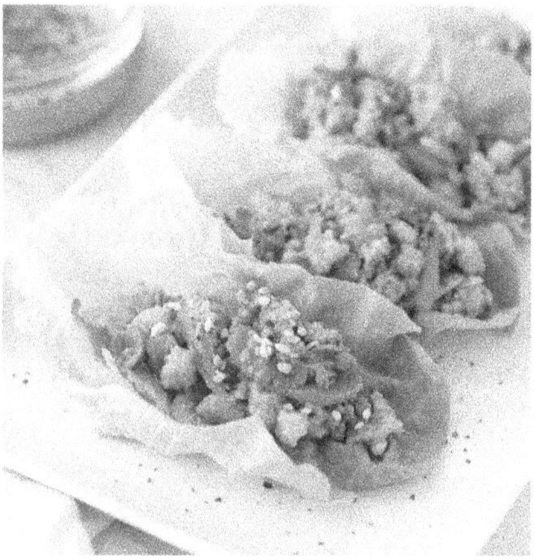

Spiced Turkey Lettuce Wraps

These turkey lettuce wraps are an easy, low-carb dinner that's full of flavor. Ground turkey is seasoned with a blend of spices, then wrapped in crisp lettuce leaves, creating a light but satisfying meal that's full of protein and anti-inflammatory goodness.

Recipe Details:

- **Servings:** 2
- **Prep Time:** 10 minutes
- **Cook Time:** 10 minutes
- **Difficulty Level:** Easy
- **Dietary Notes:** Gluten-free, dairy-free, high in protein, anti-inflammatory

Ingredients:

- 1/2 lb (225g) ground turkey
- 1 tablespoon olive oil
- 1/2 teaspoon ground cumin

- 1/2 teaspoon smoked paprika
- 1/2 teaspoon garlic powder
- 1/4 teaspoon ground cinnamon
- Salt and pepper, to taste
- 4 large lettuce leaves (such as Romaine or Butter lettuce)
- 1/4 cup diced cucumber
- 1/4 cup diced tomatoes
- Fresh cilantro for garnish

Step-by-Step Instructions:

1. Heat the olive oil in a pan over medium heat. Add the ground turkey and cook until browned, breaking it apart with a spoon as it cooks.
2. Add the cumin, smoked paprika, garlic powder, cinnamon, salt, and pepper to the turkey. Stir well to combine and cook for another 2-3 minutes.
3. While the turkey cooks, prepare the lettuce wraps. Lay the lettuce leaves flat on a plate.
4. Spoon the spiced turkey mixture into the lettuce leaves, and top with diced cucumber, diced tomatoes, and fresh cilantro.
5. Serve immediately and enjoy!

Tips and Variations:

- **Substitution:** Use ground chicken or beef if you prefer a different protein.
- **Pairing Idea:** Serve with a side of avocado or a fresh salad.
- **Variation:** Add a drizzle of tahini or a squeeze of lime for extra flavor.

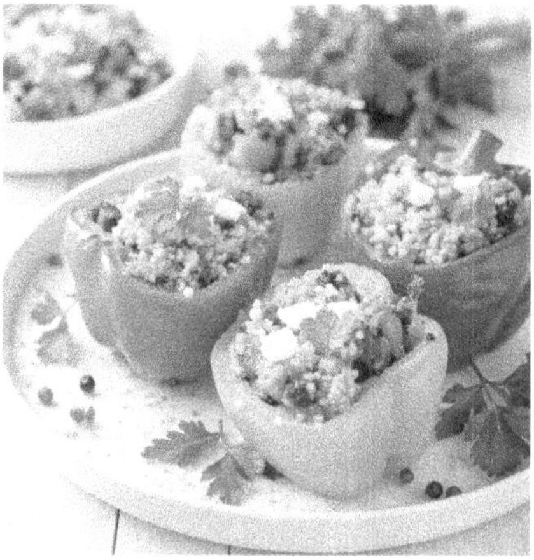

Quinoa-Stuffed Bell Peppers

These quinoa-stuffed bell peppers are a delicious and filling dinner packed with plant-based protein, fiber, and anti-inflammatory spices. The peppers are stuffed with a flavorful quinoa mixture, then baked until tender and served hot.

Recipe Details:

- **Servings:** 2
- **Prep Time:** 10 minutes
- **Cook Time:** 30 minutes
- **Difficulty Level:** Easy
- **Dietary Notes:** Gluten-free, vegan, high in fiber, anti-inflammatory

Ingredients:

- 2 large bell peppers, tops cut off and seeds removed
- 1/2 cup quinoa, rinsed
- 1 cup vegetable broth

- 1/4 cup black beans, drained and rinsed
- 1/4 cup corn kernels (fresh or frozen)
- 1/2 teaspoon ground cumin
- 1/2 teaspoon smoked paprika
- 1/4 teaspoon chili powder
- Salt and pepper, to taste

Step-by-Step Instructions:

1. Preheat your oven to 375°F (190°C).
2. In a small saucepan, combine the quinoa and vegetable broth. Bring to a boil, then cover and reduce to a simmer. Cook for 15 minutes, or until the quinoa is cooked and the liquid is absorbed.
3. Stir in the black beans, corn, cumin, smoked paprika, chili powder, salt, and pepper into the cooked quinoa.
4. Stuff each bell pepper with the quinoa mixture, packing it in tightly.
5. Place the stuffed peppers in a baking dish and cover with foil. Bake for 25-30 minutes, until the peppers are tender.
6. Serve hot, and enjoy!

Tips and Variations:

- **Substitution:** Add diced tomatoes or spinach to the quinoa stuffing for extra flavor.
- **Pairing Idea:** Serve with a simple side salad or a bowl of roasted veggies.
- **Variation:** Add a sprinkle of vegan cheese or nutritional yeast for extra flavor.

CHAPTER

5

ANTI-INFLAMMATORY SNACKS AND SIDES

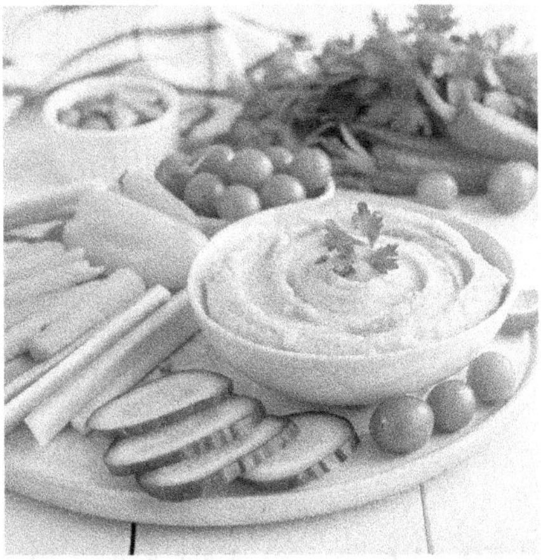

Golden Hummus with Fresh Veggies

This creamy, golden hummus is packed with the anti-inflammatory power of turmeric. Served with fresh veggies, it makes for a delicious, nutrient-packed snack that's both satisfying and full of flavor.

Recipe Details:

- **Servings:** 2
- **Prep Time:** 10 minutes
- **Cook Time:** 0 minutes
- **Difficulty Level:** Easy
- **Dietary Notes:** Gluten-free, dairy-free, vegan, high in fiber

Ingredients:

- 1 can (15 oz) chickpeas, drained and rinsed
- 2 tablespoons tahini
- 1 tablespoon olive oil
- 1 teaspoon ground turmeric

- 1/2 teaspoon ground cumin
- 1 clove garlic, minced
- 2 tablespoons lemon juice
- Salt and pepper, to taste
- Fresh vegetables (carrot sticks, cucumber, bell peppers, etc.) for dipping

Step-by-Step Instructions:

1. In a food processor, combine the chickpeas, tahini, olive oil, turmeric, cumin, garlic, lemon juice, salt, and pepper.
2. Blend until smooth, adding water as needed to reach your desired consistency.
3. Transfer the hummus to a bowl and serve with a selection of fresh, crunchy veggies for dipping.

Tips and Variations:

- **Substitution:** If you don't have tahini, you can use Greek yogurt or sunflower seed butter.
- **Pairing Idea:** Pair with whole grain crackers or a small side of quinoa for a heartier snack.
- **Variation:** Add a pinch of cayenne pepper for a spicy kick.

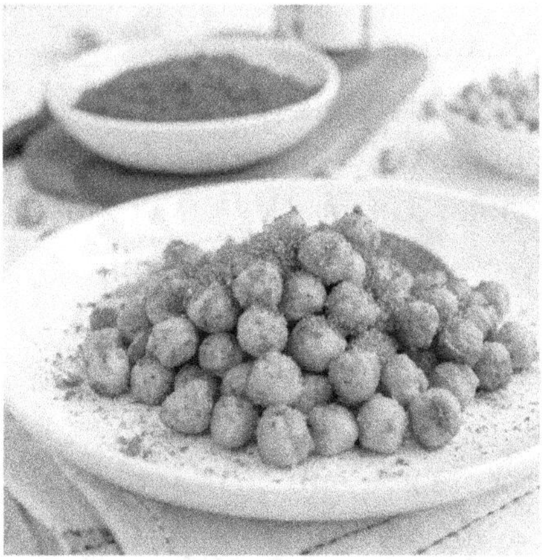

Roasted Chickpeas with Paprika

These crunchy, spiced chickpeas are the perfect healthy snack. Roasted to golden perfection with paprika and other spices, they're rich in protein, fiber, and anti-inflammatory benefits.

Recipe Details:

- **Servings:** 2
- **Prep Time:** 5 minutes
- **Cook Time:** 25 minutes
- **Difficulty Level:** Easy
- **Dietary Notes:** Gluten-free, dairy-free, vegan, high in protein

Ingredients:

- 1 can (15 oz) chickpeas, drained, rinsed, and patted dry
- 1 tablespoon olive oil
- 1 teaspoon smoked paprika
- 1/2 teaspoon garlic powder

- 1/4 teaspoon ground turmeric
- Salt and pepper, to taste

Step-by-Step Instructions:

1. Preheat your oven to 400°F (200°C).
2. In a bowl, toss the chickpeas with olive oil, smoked paprika, garlic powder, turmeric, salt, and pepper.
3. Spread the chickpeas in a single layer on a baking sheet.
4. Roast in the oven for 25 minutes, shaking the pan halfway through to ensure even cooking, until crispy and golden.
5. Let cool for a few minutes before serving.

Tips and Variations:

- **Substitution:** Add your favorite spices, such as cayenne pepper for heat or rosemary for an herbal twist.
- **Pairing Idea:** Serve with a side of guacamole or hummus for a satisfying snack spread.
- **Variation:** For a sweet version, drizzle with a bit of honey or maple syrup and a sprinkle of cinnamon before roasting.

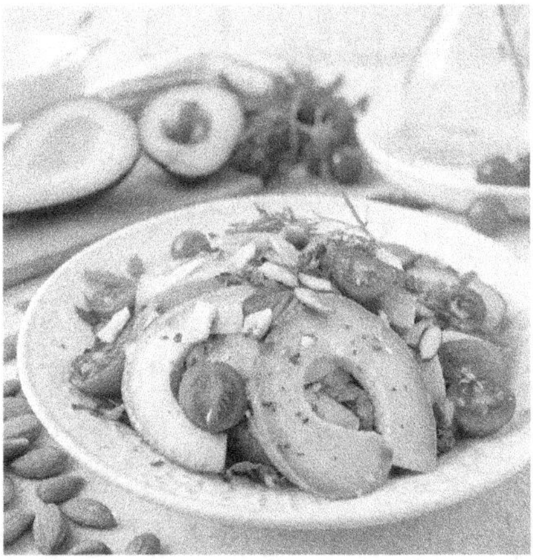

Avocado and Cucumber Salad

This refreshing salad combines creamy avocado with crunchy cucumber, all tossed in a light, tangy dressing. The combination of healthy fats and anti-inflammatory cucumbers makes it a perfect, refreshing side dish.

Recipe Details:

- **Servings:** 2
- **Prep Time:** 5 minutes
- **Cook Time:** 0 minutes
- **Difficulty Level:** Easy
- **Dietary Notes:** Gluten-free, dairy-free, vegan, anti-inflammatory

Ingredients:

- 1 ripe avocado, diced
- 1 cucumber, sliced
- 1 tablespoon olive oil

- 1 tablespoon apple cider vinegar
- 1 teaspoon lemon juice
- Salt and pepper, to taste
- Fresh parsley or cilantro for garnish

Step-by-Step Instructions:

1. In a bowl, combine the diced avocado and sliced cucumber.
2. In a small bowl, whisk together the olive oil, apple cider vinegar, lemon juice, salt, and pepper.
3. Drizzle the dressing over the avocado and cucumber, then toss gently to combine.
4. Garnish with fresh parsley or cilantro and serve immediately.

Tips and Variations:

- **Substitution:** Add cherry tomatoes, red onion, or a sprinkle of hemp seeds for extra texture and flavor.
- **Pairing Idea:** Serve with grilled fish or chicken for a light, balanced meal.
- **Variation:** Add a teaspoon of chia seeds for a fiber boost.

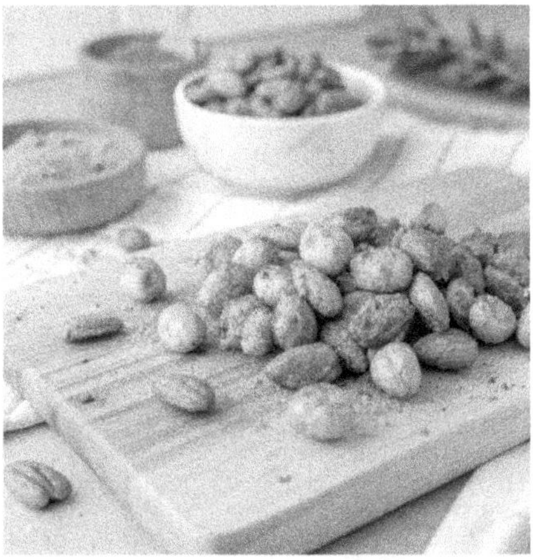

Turmeric Roasted Nuts

These turmeric roasted nuts are a delicious and crunchy snack that combines the anti-inflammatory power of turmeric with the healthy fats from almonds and cashews. Perfect for snacking or adding to salads.

Recipe Details:

- **Servings:** 2
- **Prep Time:** 5 minutes
- **Cook Time:** 15 minutes
- **Difficulty Level:** Easy
- **Dietary Notes:** Gluten-free, dairy-free, vegan, high in healthy fats

Ingredients:

- 1 cup mixed nuts (almonds, cashews, walnuts)
- 1 tablespoon olive oil
- 1 teaspoon ground turmeric

- 1/2 teaspoon garlic powder
- Salt and pepper, to taste

Step-by-Step Instructions:

1. Preheat your oven to 350°F (175°C).
2. In a bowl, toss the mixed nuts with olive oil, turmeric, garlic powder, salt, and pepper.
3. Spread the nuts in a single layer on a baking sheet.
4. Roast in the oven for 12-15 minutes, stirring once halfway through, until golden and fragrant.
5. Let cool before serving.

Tips and Variations:

- **Substitution:** Use any combination of your favorite nuts or add seeds like sunflower or pumpkin.
- **Pairing Idea:** Enjoy with a glass of herbal tea or as a topping for a salad or grain bowl.
- **Variation:** Add a pinch of cayenne pepper or smoked paprika for extra flavor.

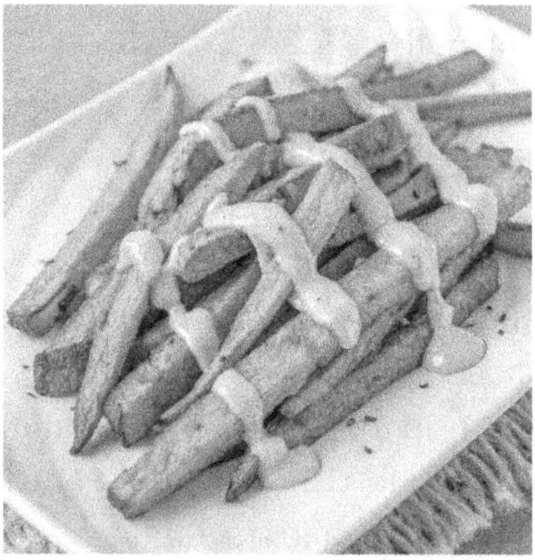

Sweet Potato Fries with Tahini Drizzle

These crispy sweet potato fries are baked to perfection and topped with a creamy tahini drizzle. Not only are they delicious, but sweet potatoes are also full of anti-inflammatory benefits, making this snack both satisfying and healing.

Recipe Details:

- **Servings:** 2
- **Prep Time:** 10 minutes
- **Cook Time:** 25 minutes
- **Difficulty Level:** Easy
- **Dietary Notes:** Gluten-free, dairy-free, vegan, high in vitamin A and fiber

Ingredients:

- 2 medium sweet potatoes, cut into fries
- 2 tablespoons olive oil
- 1 teaspoon smoked paprika

- 1/2 teaspoon garlic powder
- Salt and pepper, to taste

For the Tahini Drizzle:

- 2 tablespoons tahini
- 1 tablespoon lemon juice
- 1 teaspoon maple syrup
- Water, as needed to thin

Step-by-Step Instructions:

1. Preheat your oven to 400°F (200°C).
2. Toss the sweet potato fries with olive oil, smoked paprika, garlic powder, salt, and pepper.
3. Spread the fries in a single layer on a baking sheet and bake for 20-25 minutes, flipping halfway through, until golden and crispy.
4. While the fries bake, whisk together the tahini, lemon juice, maple syrup, and a splash of water to reach a smooth, drizzle-able consistency.
5. Serve the sweet potato fries with a drizzle of tahini sauce on top.

Tips and Variations:

- **Substitution:** Add a sprinkle of chili flakes or cumin to the fries for extra flavor.
- **Pairing Idea:** Serve with a side of greens or a protein-rich dip like hummus.
- **Variation:** Top with a handful of chopped parsley for a fresh, herby touch.

CHAPTER

6

SOOTHING DRINKS AND HEALING TREATS

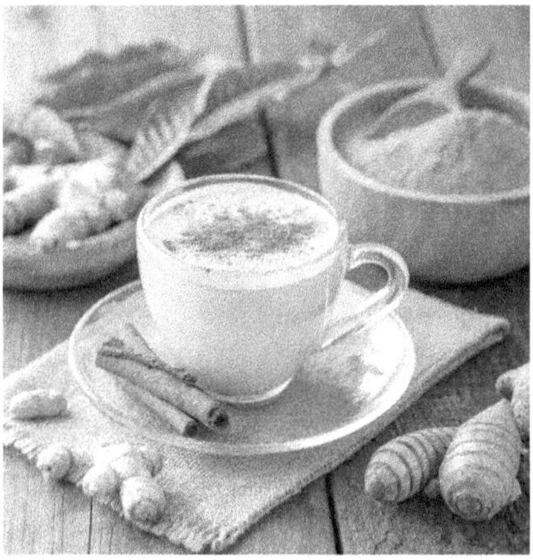

Ginger-Turmeric Tea

This warming, golden tea combines the anti-inflammatory properties of ginger and turmeric, making it an ideal drink to soothe the body and calm inflammation. Perfect for sipping any time of day to reduce pain and discomfort.

Recipe Details:

- **Servings:** 2
- **Prep Time:** 5 minutes
- **Cook Time:** 10 minutes
- **Difficulty Level:** Easy
- **Dietary Notes:** Gluten-free, dairy-free, vegan, anti-inflammatory

Ingredients:

- 2 cups water
- 1-inch piece of fresh ginger, peeled and sliced

- 1-inch piece of fresh turmeric, peeled and sliced (or 1 teaspoon ground turmeric)
- 1 teaspoon honey (optional)
- 1 tablespoon lemon juice
- A pinch of black pepper (to increase turmeric absorption)

Step-by-Step Instructions:

1. In a small saucepan, bring the water to a boil.
2. Add the ginger and turmeric slices (or ground turmeric) to the water and let it simmer for about 10 minutes.
3. Strain the tea into mugs.
4. Stir in honey and lemon juice to taste, then add a pinch of black pepper.
5. Enjoy the soothing, anti-inflammatory benefits of your ginger-turmeric tea!

Tips and Variations:

- **Substitution:** You can use ginger powder and turmeric powder if fresh root is unavailable.
- **Pairing Idea:** Pair with a light snack, such as an avocado toast or a handful of nuts.
- **Variation:** Add a pinch of cayenne pepper for a spicier kick.

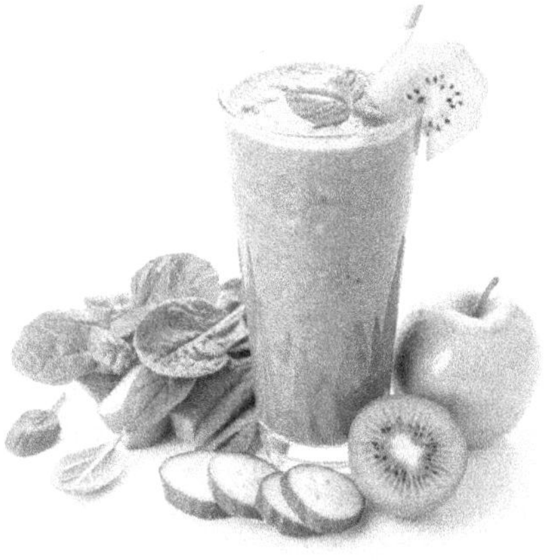

Anti-Inflammatory Green Smoothie

This green smoothie is loaded with anti-inflammatory ingredients like spinach, flaxseeds, and ginger. It's perfect for starting your day or as a refreshing, nutrient-packed snack.

Recipe Details:

- **Servings:** 2
- **Prep Time:** 5 minutes
- **Cook Time:** 0 minutes
- **Difficulty Level:** Easy
- **Dietary Notes:** Gluten-free, dairy-free, vegan, high in fiber

Ingredients:

- 1 cup spinach
- 1/2 banana
- 1/2 cup frozen pineapple
- 1/2 teaspoon grated fresh ginger
- 1 tablespoon ground flaxseeds

- 1/2 cup unsweetened almond milk (or any preferred milk)
- 1/2 cup water (optional, for thinning)
- Ice cubes (optional, for a thicker smoothie)

Step-by-Step Instructions:

1. Add all ingredients to a blender: spinach, banana, pineapple, ginger, flaxseeds, almond milk, and water (if using).
2. Blend until smooth, adding more liquid if needed to reach your desired consistency.
3. Pour into glasses and enjoy immediately!

Tips and Variations:

- **Substitution:** Swap spinach for kale or arugula for a different flavor.
- **Pairing Idea:** Serve with a handful of mixed nuts or a protein-packed granola.
- **Variation:** Add a scoop of plant-based protein powder for an extra boost.

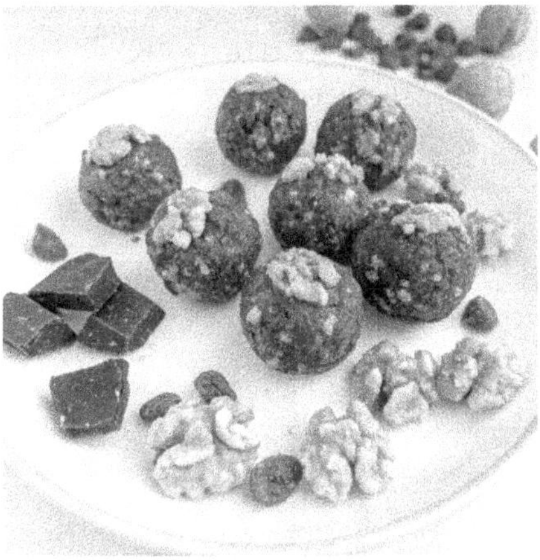

Dark Chocolate and Walnut Energy Bites

These energy bites combine the richness of dark chocolate with the crunch of walnuts, offering a satisfying snack that's both delicious and anti-inflammatory. Perfect for an on-the-go pick-me-up.

Recipe Details:

- **Servings:** 8-10 bites
- **Prep Time:** 10 minutes
- **Cook Time:** 0 minutes
- **Difficulty Level:** Easy
- **Dietary Notes:** Gluten-free, dairy-free, vegan, high in healthy fats

Ingredients:

- 1/2 cup walnuts
- 1/4 cup dark chocolate chips (70% cocoa or higher)
- 1/4 cup almond butter

- 1 tablespoon chia seeds
- 2 tablespoons maple syrup or honey
- 1/2 teaspoon vanilla extract
- A pinch of salt

Step-by-Step Instructions:

1. In a food processor, combine the walnuts, dark chocolate chips, almond butter, chia seeds, maple syrup (or honey), vanilla extract, and salt.
2. Pulse until everything is finely chopped and well-combined.
3. Scoop the mixture into small balls (about 1 inch in diameter) and roll them between your hands.
4. Place on a parchment-lined tray and refrigerate for at least 30 minutes before serving.

Tips and Variations:

- **Substitution:** Use any nut butter you prefer, such as peanut or cashew butter.
- **Pairing Idea:** Serve these bites with a hot cup of ginger-turmeric tea or a glass of almond milk.
- **Variation:** Add a pinch of cinnamon or nutmeg for added warmth.

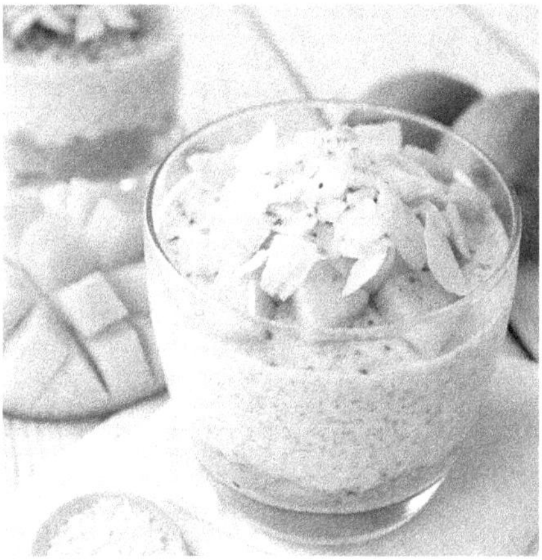

Chia Seed Pudding with Coconut and Mango

This creamy chia seed pudding is topped with sweet mango and coconut, making for a refreshing, anti-inflammatory treat. Chia seeds are rich in omega-3s, and the tropical flavors of mango and coconut will make it feel like a treat.

Recipe Details:

- **Servings:** 2
- **Prep Time:** 5 minutes
- **Cook Time:** 0 minutes
- **Difficulty Level:** Easy
- **Dietary Notes:** Gluten-free, dairy-free, vegan, high in omega-3s

Ingredients:

- 1/2 cup chia seeds
- 1 cup coconut milk (or any preferred milk)
- 1 tablespoon maple syrup or honey

- 1/2 teaspoon vanilla extract
- 1/2 mango, diced
- 2 tablespoons shredded coconut

Step-by-Step Instructions:

1. In a bowl, mix the chia seeds, coconut milk, maple syrup (or honey), and vanilla extract.
2. Stir well to combine and let sit for 5 minutes. Stir again to prevent clumping.
3. Cover the bowl and refrigerate for at least 2 hours or overnight, until the pudding has thickened.
4. Before serving, top with diced mango and shredded coconut.

Tips and Variations:

- **Substitution:** You can use almond milk or oat milk if you don't prefer coconut milk.
- **Pairing Idea:** Enjoy with a small handful of almonds or walnuts for extra crunch.
- **Variation:** Add a sprinkle of cinnamon or cardamom for an extra layer of flavor.

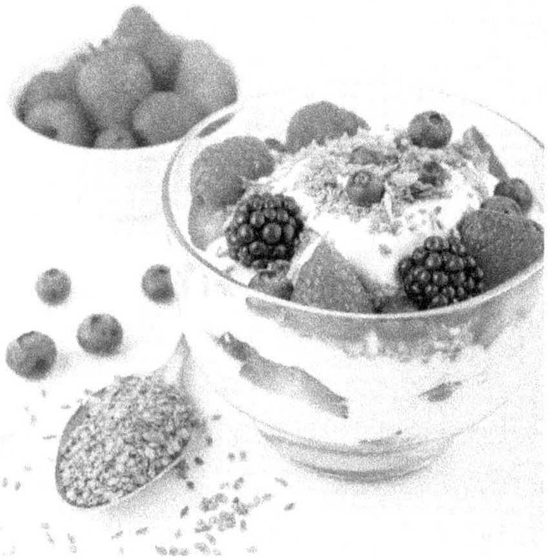

Berry and Yogurt Parfait with Flaxseed

This simple yet delicious parfait is made with layers of creamy yogurt, fresh berries, and a sprinkle of ground flaxseed. It's not only a treat for your taste buds but also an anti-inflammatory powerhouse thanks to the antioxidants in the berries and the omega-3s in the flaxseed.

Recipe Details:

- **Servings:** 2
- **Prep Time:** 5 minutes
- **Cook Time:** 0 minutes
- **Difficulty Level:** Easy
- **Dietary Notes:** Gluten-free, dairy-free (if using plant-based yogurt), high in fiber

Ingredients:

- 1 cup plain Greek yogurt (or plant-based yogurt)

- 1/2 cup mixed berries (blueberries, raspberries, strawberries)
- 1 tablespoon ground flaxseed
- 1 tablespoon honey or maple syrup (optional)
- A handful of granola or nuts for topping (optional)

Step-by-Step Instructions:

1. In serving glasses or bowls, layer the Greek yogurt and mixed berries.
2. Drizzle with honey or maple syrup (if desired).
3. Sprinkle ground flaxseed on top.
4. Top with granola or chopped nuts for added crunch.
5. Serve immediately or refrigerate until ready to enjoy.

Tips and Variations:

- **Substitution:** Use any combination of berries you prefer, or add sliced banana for more variety.
- **Pairing Idea:** Pair with a refreshing green smoothie for a filling breakfast or snack.
- **Variation:** Add a spoonful of almond butter or peanut butter for extra protein.

CHAPTER

7

2-WEEK ANTI-INFLAMMATORY MEAL PLAN

Ready to start reducing inflammation while enjoying a variety of nourishing meals? This 2-week meal plan is designed to be simple, convenient, and effective. Every meal is crafted with anti-inflammatory ingredients to keep your body feeling its best, without compromising on flavor. Whether you're new to meal prepping or a seasoned pro, these meals are quick, easy, and great for your health.

What You'll Find in This Chapter:

- **Ready-to-Follow Weekly Plans with Balanced Meals:** Each meal is carefully crafted to offer anti-inflammatory benefits while keeping things balanced with proteins, healthy fats, and plenty of veggies.

- **Shopping Lists for Ease and Convenience:** We've organized the shopping lists so that you can easily stock your kitchen with all the ingredients you'll need for each week.
- **Prep Tips for Saving Time and Staying Consistent:** Meal prepping doesn't have to be overwhelming. These tips will help you stay on track and save valuable time throughout your busy week.

Week 1: Anti-Inflammatory Meal Plan

Day	Breakfast	Lunch	Dinner	Snack
Monday	Turmeric Scrambled Eggs with Spinach and Avocado	Quinoa Salad with Chickpeas and Cucumbers	Grilled Salmon with Roasted Veggies and Sweet Potato	Handful of Walnuts and Turmeric Tea
Tuesday	Chia Seed Pudding with Berries and Flaxseed	Mediterranean Hummus and Veggie Wrap	Chicken Stir-fry with Broccoli, Bell Peppers, and Brown Rice	Carrot and Cucumber Sticks with Guacamole
Wednesday	Green Smoothie (Spinach, Ginger, Banana)	Roasted Veggie Bowl with Lentils and Tahini Dressing	Baked Chicken Thighs with Sweet Potatoes and Greens	Apple Slices with Almond Butter
Thursday	Overnight Oats with Chia and Blueberries	Avocado Toast with a Side of Mixed Greens	Grilled Turkey Burgers with Roasted Asparagus	Handful of Almonds and Lemon-Infused Water
Friday	Veggie Omelette with Mushrooms and Spinach	Quinoa and Black Bean Salad with Lime Vinaigrette	Shrimp Stir-fry with Kale and Cauliflower Rice	Roasted Chickpeas with Paprika
Saturday	Porridge with Almond Butter and Cinnamon	Grilled Chicken Salad with Olive Oil Dressing	Baked Cod with Brussels Sprouts and Quinoa	A handful of Mixed Berries with a sprinkle of Flaxseed

Day	Breakfast	Lunch	Dinner	Snack
Sunday	Sweet Potato Hash with Eggs and Avocado	Zucchini Noodles with Pesto and Cherry Tomatoes	Beef and Veggie Skewers with a Side of Couscous	Celery Sticks with Peanut Butter

Week 2: Anti-Inflammatory Meal Plan

Day	Breakfast	Lunch	Dinner	Snack
Monday	Avocado Toast with a Boiled Egg and Tomato	Grilled Chicken Wrap with Hummus and Veggies	Grilled Salmon with Broccoli and Quinoa	Handful of Walnuts and Ginger-Turmeric Tea
Tuesday	Smoothie Bowl with Berries, Chia, and Almonds	Spinach and Feta Salad with Olive Oil Dressing	Stir-Fried Shrimp with Cauliflower Rice	Carrot and Cucumber Sticks with Hummus
Wednesday	Scrambled Eggs with Spinach and Mushrooms	Grilled Veggie Salad with Tahini Dressing	Turkey Meatballs with Zucchini Noodles	A handful of Mixed Nuts and a Green Tea
Thursday	Porridge with Chia, Flaxseeds, and Berries	Chicken Avocado Salad with Olive Oil Dressing	Beef Stir-fry with Sweet Potato and Spinach	Apple Slices with Almond Butter
Friday	Green Smoothie with Kale, Banana, and Almond Milk	Tuna Salad with Mixed Greens and Olive Oil	Grilled Chicken with Roasted Veggies	Roasted Chickpeas with Sea Salt
Saturday	Coconut Yogurt with Chia, Almonds, and Berries	Lentil Soup with a Side Salad	Grilled Shrimp with Zucchini and Brown Rice	Handful of Almonds and Carrot Sticks
Sunday	Scrambled Tofu with Spinach and Avocado	Quinoa Salad with Roasted Veggies and Chickpeas	Baked Cod with Brussels Sprouts and Sweet Potatoes	Fresh Mango Slices and a Handful of Cashews

Shopping Lists for Each Week

To make your grocery shopping stress-free, here's a handy shopping list to ensure you have everything you need for each week.

Week 1 Shopping List:

- **Proteins:**
  - Eggs (1 dozen)
  - Salmon (2 fillets)
  - Chicken thighs (4 pieces)
  - Canned chickpeas (2 cans)
  - Quinoa (1 bag)
  - Chicken breast (2 pieces)
  - Turkey (1 lb)
  - Cod fillets (2 pieces)
- **Vegetables:**
  - Spinach (2 bags)
  - Avocados (4)
  - Bell peppers (2)
  - Sweet potatoes (4)
  - Broccoli (2 crowns)
  - Brussels sprouts (1 lb)
  - Mushrooms (1 pack)
  - Cucumber (2)
  - Kale (1 bunch)
  - Asparagus (1 bunch)
- **Fruits:**
  - Mixed berries (frozen or fresh)

  - Apples (4)
  - Lemons (2)
- **Grains & Legumes:**
  - Brown rice (1 bag)
  - Lentils (1 bag)
  - Black beans (1 can)
  - Quinoa (1 bag)
- **Nuts & Seeds:**
  - Walnuts (1 bag)
  - Almond butter (1 jar)
  - Flaxseed (1 bag)
  - Chia seeds (1 bag)
  - Almonds (1 bag)
- **Dairy & Dairy Alternatives:**
  - Plain Greek yogurt (1 tub)
  - Coconut milk (1 can)
- **Oils & Condiments:**
  - Olive oil (1 bottle)
  - Tahini (1 jar)
  - Apple cider vinegar (1 bottle)
  - Honey (1 jar)

Week 2 Shopping List:

- **Proteins:**
    - Eggs (1 dozen)
    - Chicken breast (2 pieces)
    - Shrimp (1 lb)
    - Ground turkey (1 lb)
    - Canned tuna (2 cans)
    - Salmon fillets (2 pieces)
- **Vegetables:**
    - Spinach (2 bags)
    - Zucchini (3)
    - Sweet potatoes (4)
    - Broccoli (2 crowns)
    - Bell peppers (2)
    - Asparagus (1 bunch)
    - Mushrooms (1 pack)
    - Carrots (1 bag)
    - Mixed greens (1 bag)
    - Kale (1 bunch)
- **Fruits:**
    - Mixed berries (frozen or fresh)
    - Bananas (2)
    - Apples (4)
    - Avocados (4)
    - Mango (1)
- **Grains & Legumes:**
    - Quinoa (1 bag)

  - Cauliflower rice (1 bag)
  - Lentils (1 bag)
- **Nuts & Seeds:**
  - Almonds (1 bag)
  - Flaxseed (1 bag)
  - Chia seeds (1 bag)
  - Cashews (1 bag)
- **Dairy & Dairy Alternatives:**
  - Plant-based yogurt (1 tub)
  - Coconut yogurt (1 tub)
- **Oils & Condiments:**
  - Olive oil (1 bottle)
  - Tahini (1 jar)
  - Maple syrup (1 bottle)
  - Vinegar (apple cider or balsamic)

Prep Tips for Saving Time and Staying Consistent:

1. **Batch Cook:** Cook your grains (like quinoa and brown rice) and beans (such as chickpeas and black beans) in bulk at the beginning of the week. This will save you time during the day, allowing you to focus on other meals.
2. **Pre-Cut Veggies:** Wash and chop vegetables in advance, storing them in airtight containers to keep them fresh. Pre-cut veggies will make it easy to assemble salads, stir-fries, and snacks on the go.
3. **Snack Prep:** Portion out snacks like nuts, seeds, and fresh fruit for easy grab-and-go options. Having them ready will prevent you from reaching for something less healthy.
4. **Cook Once, Eat Twice:** Prepare extra servings of dinner so that you have leftovers for lunch the following day. This

helps with consistency and reduces the time spent cooking each day.

CHAPTER

8

TROUBLESHOOTING AND STAYING ON TRACK

Embarking on a new anti-inflammatory diet can feel like a big step, but don't worry—you're not alone. Just like any new lifestyle change, there will be some bumps along the way. The key is to understand the common challenges that come up and to have simple solutions ready so you can stay on track. I've included tips on how to overcome those obstacles, as well as ways to keep things manageable, affordable, and motivating so that you can continue seeing the results you're after.

Let's dive in!

Common Challenges and Simple Solutions

1. Challenge: Lack of Time for Meal Prep

Life is busy, and it's easy to fall into the trap of saying, "I don't have time to cook." But here's the thing: meal prepping doesn't have to take hours. It's all about working smarter, not harder.

Solution:

- **Batch Cooking:** Cook large portions of grains (like quinoa or rice), legumes (like beans or lentils), and protein (like chicken or salmon) in one go. Store them in the fridge or freezer, so you always have meals ready to go.
- **One-Pan Meals:** Simplify cooking by making meals that only require one pan. Think sheet-pan chicken with veggies or stir-fries that come together in minutes.
- **Prep Ingredients Ahead:** Chop veggies, wash greens, or pre-cook certain elements of your meal the night before or during your downtime on weekends. This will save you time during the week when you're feeling rushed.

2. Challenge: Staying on Track with Snacking

Sometimes the temptation to snack on something processed or sugary is too strong, especially when you're busy or feeling tired.

Solution:

- **Healthy Snacks in Reach:** Stock up on anti-inflammatory snacks like raw nuts, seeds, fresh fruits, and veggies. Having them on hand makes it easier to grab something that aligns with your goals.
- **Plan Snacks Ahead:** Try adding a quick, healthy snack to your meal plan, like almond butter with apple slices or a handful of roasted chickpeas. Pre-pack snacks so you don't end up grabbing something unhealthy.
- **Drink More Water:** Sometimes thirst is mistaken for hunger. Staying hydrated throughout the day can reduce unnecessary snacking and cravings.

3. Challenge: Overcoming Cravings for Unhealthy Foods

Whether it's a craving for chocolate, chips, or pizza, we all have those moments when we want to indulge.

Solution:

- **Substitute, Don't Deprive:** Instead of trying to eliminate all your favorite foods, find anti-inflammatory substitutes. For instance, swap regular pasta with zucchini noodles, or try dark chocolate with a high cocoa percentage when you need a sweet treat.
- **Embrace Healthy Fats:** Healthy fats (like avocado, olive oil, and coconut oil) help curb cravings and keep you feeling full. Adding them to your meals ensures you don't feel deprived.
- **Mindful Eating:** Take a moment before you eat to check in with yourself. Are you truly hungry, or is it just a craving? Often, slowing down helps us reconnect with what our body actually needs.

How to Keep It Affordable and Manageable

Eating an anti-inflammatory diet doesn't have to break the bank. With some smart shopping strategies, it's entirely possible to keep costs low while fueling your body with the right foods.

1. Plan Your Meals:

Meal planning doesn't just help with staying on track—it also helps save money. When you plan your meals in advance, you can buy in bulk, avoid food waste, and make sure you only purchase what you need. If you're following the meal plans from the previous chapters, you already have a head start!

2. Shop in Season:

Seasonal produce is typically cheaper and fresher. By buying fruits and vegetables that are in season, you can save money while eating more flavorful, nutrient-dense meals. For example, root vegetables like carrots, sweet potatoes, and squash are often more affordable during colder months.

3. Buy Frozen Produce:

Frozen fruits and vegetables are just as nutritious as fresh and can be more affordable, especially for out-of-season items. Plus, they last longer, which means less waste.

4. Focus on Whole Foods:

Processed foods might seem cheaper upfront, but they're often filled with hidden sugars, unhealthy fats, and additives. Whole foods, like fresh vegetables, fruits, whole grains, and lean proteins, are the foundation of a healthy anti-inflammatory diet—and they're often more budget-friendly when purchased in bulk.

5. Use Leftovers Creatively:

Repurpose leftovers to create new meals. Leftover roasted chicken can be turned into chicken salad, and roasted vegetables can be repurposed into a soup or salad the next day. Get creative to make sure nothing goes to waste!

Staying Motivated and Seeing Results

It's easy to feel overwhelmed in the beginning, especially when you're adjusting to a new diet. But trust me—results are worth it! It may take a few weeks to notice physical changes, but the mental clarity, increased energy, and reduced inflammation will begin to show.

1. Track Your Progress:

Keep a journal or take photos of your meals and how you feel each day. It's easy to forget the progress you've made, so when you look back at your journey, you'll realize just how far you've come.

2. Celebrate Small Wins:

The journey to healing your body is a process, so celebrate every milestone along the way. Did you make it through the week without indulging in unhealthy snacks? That's a win! Did you meal prep for the week? Celebrate that! Each step forward counts.

3. Surround Yourself with Support:

It's much easier to stay motivated when you have a support system. Whether it's a friend, family member, or online community, being able to share your experiences and lean on others when you're feeling stuck can keep you moving forward.

4. Be Kind to Yourself:

If you slip up, don't be hard on yourself. The anti-inflammatory lifestyle is about making better choices most of the time, not perfection. Allow yourself some grace and get back on track. Rome wasn't built in a day—and neither is a new eating habit.

Adapting Recipes for Dietary Needs (Gluten-Free, Dairy-Free, etc.)

Whether you have specific dietary restrictions or just prefer to avoid certain foods, adapting recipes to fit your needs is easier than you might think.

1. Gluten-Free Substitutes:

- **Flours:** Use almond flour or coconut flour instead of regular flour in baking recipes.
- **Pasta:** Substitute gluten-containing pasta with zucchini noodles or gluten-free pasta options made from rice, quinoa, or chickpeas.
- **Bread:** Opt for gluten-free bread or use lettuce wraps for sandwiches.

2. Dairy-Free Alternatives:

- **Milk and Cream:** Almond milk, coconut milk, and oat milk are excellent substitutes for dairy milk in smoothies, coffee, or baking.

- **Cheese:** Nutritional yeast, cashew-based cheese, or dairy-free cheeses made from coconut are great substitutes for regular cheese in salads and pasta dishes.
- **Yogurt:** Coconut-based or almond-based yogurt is a perfect option for dairy-free breakfasts or snacks.

3. Nut-Free Substitutes:

- **Nut Butter:** If you're avoiding nuts, sunflower seed butter or pumpkin seed butter are great options for smoothies, oatmeal, or snacks.
- **Milk Alternatives:** Instead of almond milk, go for oat milk or coconut milk.

4. Low-Sugar Options: If you're looking to cut back on sugar, swap regular sweeteners with natural options like stevia, monk fruit, or erythritol. Always be mindful of portion sizes to ensure you're not overdoing it.

5. Paleo Modifications: If you're following a paleo diet, swap out quinoa and legumes with extra vegetables and healthy fats like avocado, coconut oil, or nuts (if you can tolerate them).

The beauty of this anti-inflammatory lifestyle is its flexibility. With simple ingredient swaps, you can adapt every recipe to suit your needs without compromising on flavor or nutrition.

Staying on track with your anti-inflammatory journey might seem challenging at times, but with a bit of preparation and the right mindset, it's completely doable. Remember, small changes lead to big results, so take it one step at a time, and trust in the process. You've got this!

CONCLUSION

First of all, congratulations! You've made it to the end of this book, and that's no small feat. Whether you're just starting out or have been following the anti-inflammatory diet for a while, I want you to take a moment to celebrate yourself for making it this far. Changing the way we eat and care for our bodies is one of the most powerful things we can do for our health—and you've already taken a huge step in the right direction.

But this is just the beginning of your journey to better health. It might seem overwhelming at times, but with the tools and knowledge you now have, you can confidently continue on your path toward healing. It's not about perfection; it's about making healthier choices, staying consistent, and trusting that each step you take is bringing you closer to feeling your best.

Let's dive into a few important ways to help you stay on track, celebrate your progress, and build lasting, healthy habits.

Celebrating Your Progress

One of the most important things to remember as you continue your journey is to take time to celebrate your progress—no matter how big or small. If you've noticed a reduction in inflammation, increased energy, better digestion, or clearer skin, those are huge wins! These changes are the results of your dedication, and they deserve to be acknowledged.

Here are a few ways to celebrate your progress:

- **Take photos:** Snap pictures of your meals, your body, or any changes you notice over time. You may not notice the small changes day by day, but looking back at photos can be a great way to track your journey.
- **Write in a journal:** Keep a record of how you're feeling—physically, mentally, and emotionally. It's easy to forget how far you've come, but journaling will help remind you of your growth and achievements.
- **Treat yourself to something non-food related:** Maybe you buy yourself a new workout outfit, enjoy a relaxing bath, or indulge in a hobby you love. Celebrating doesn't have to involve food—it can be a way to reward yourself with something that nurtures your overall well-being.

Remember, this journey is about healing your body, not about striving for perfection. So, every step you take is a reason to be proud!

Building Long-Term Healthy Habits

The real magic happens when you build long-term habits that support your health and well-being. Sustainable change doesn't happen overnight—it's a gradual process. As you continue to implement the strategies you've learned here, aim to focus on creating habits that are realistic, achievable, and nourishing.

Here are a few strategies for building lasting habits:

- **Start small:** The key to lasting change is starting small and adding more over time. Begin with a few key habits, like eating anti-inflammatory meals consistently or drinking more water each day. Once these habits become second nature, you can build on them.

- **Be patient with yourself:** There will be days when things don't go as planned, and that's okay. Building healthy habits is a process, and it's important to be patient and kind to yourself when challenges arise. Perfection isn't the goal—progress is.
- **Track your habits:** Whether you use an app or a physical journal, tracking your meals, symptoms, and habits can help you stay on track. It will also give you valuable insight into what's working and what might need adjusting.
- **Make it a lifestyle:** The anti-inflammatory way of eating isn't a temporary diet—it's a lifestyle. Treat it as such. Focus on nourishing your body every day, and make it part of your routine. Soon, healthy habits will feel like second nature.

By building these habits, you'll find that this way of eating no longer feels like a "diet" but rather a sustainable, long-term approach to feeling better every day.

Additional Resources and Support

As you continue on your anti-inflammatory journey, know that you don't have to do it alone. There are plenty of resources out there to support you along the way, whether you're looking for recipe ideas, more in-depth advice, or a community of like-minded individuals. Here are some resources to help you stay motivated and informed:

1. Online Communities:

Find online forums, Facebook groups, or Instagram accounts that focus on the anti-inflammatory lifestyle. These communities are filled with people who share their own experiences, recipes, and tips to keep you inspired.

2. Blogs and Websites:

Many experts share their knowledge online about anti-inflammatory eating and its benefits. Check out reputable blogs and websites for more recipes, research, and advice.

3. Apps:

There are several apps designed to track your meals, symptoms, and progress. Apps like MyFitnessPal or Yummly can help you stay on top of your meals and offer new recipe ideas when you need them.

4. Cookbooks:

This book is just the beginning! There are plenty of other anti-inflammatory cookbooks available that dive deeper into specific foods, health conditions, or recipes for different dietary needs.

5. Your Doctor or Nutritionist:

If you're struggling with any health issues or just want more personalized guidance, don't hesitate to reach out to your healthcare provider. They can offer tailored advice and resources specific to your needs.

Final Thoughts

The road to better health is a journey—and, like any journey, it will have its twists and turns. But as long as you stay consistent, continue celebrating your progress, and trust in the power of nourishing your body with anti-inflammatory foods, you'll see the results. Your health is in your hands, and every positive choice you make is a step toward living a healthier, happier life.

Now, it's time to embrace the new you. I believe in you and your ability to make lasting, positive changes. The work you're putting into your health today will pay off in so many ways in the years to come.

You've got this!